DIETS TO HELP CATARRH

The eliminative diet given here can banish the miseries of catarrh by reducing the formation of mucus and stimulating the expulsion of waste products. Also includes advice on correct breathing, hydropathic (water) treatments and steam treatment.

GW00375133

DIETS TO HELP

CATARRH

by

ALAN MOYLE
N.D., M.B.N.O.A.

THORSONS PUBLISHERS LIMITED
Wellingborough, Northamptonshire.

First published 1970
Second Impression 1974
Third Impression 1977

ISBN 0 7225 0155 2

*Made and Printed in Great Britain by
Weatherby Woolnough Ltd., Wellingborough
Northants, England*

CONTENTS

CHAPTER ONE

HOW CATARRH STARTS

CATARRH is the term commonly associated with irritation of the mucous membranes, especially of the air passages, and an accumulation of mucus which has to be constantly cleared from the throat and nasal passages. The same condition in varying degrees can arise, however, wherever mucous membranes are situated and can be inflamed and irritated.

The extent to which catarrh can attack the system can be gauged by the extent of mucous membrane itself. This membrane lines the respiratory tract, the alimentary tract and parts of the genito-urinary system.

Mucous membrane is one of a layer of specialized cells which line the cavities of the body. The membranes all secrete a fluid to lubricate or moisten the cavity they line. Mucous membrane produces mucus.

The membrane is made up of a special type of cell which, in certain parts, for example the trachea (windpipe), has minute lash-like projections which maintain the free movement of fluid over the membrane. The cells in the mucous membrane are closely packed and those which become distended with mucous secretion are termed goblet cells. It is these cells which become more and more distended and finally rupture, discharging the secretion on to the surface of the membranous lining. The mucus, which is the secretion of the membrane, is composed of water, salts and a protein called mucin. The secretion is sticky, a fact well known to the victim of nasal or bronchial catarrh.

When mucous membrane is irritated, more mucus is formed and it is this excessive production of mucus which creates a catarrhal condition. It is not surprising, therefore, considering mucous membrane extends so far through the body that catarrh can be a widespread source of trouble. While catarrh is commonly associated with bronchitis, chills, and diseases of the respiratory system, it is also the cause of some digestive disorders, diarrhoea, colitis, and cystitis and, of course, catarrhal deafness. Indeed, catarrh is a very common cause of deafness.

Catarrh is not a dramatic disease. Possibly for this reason, and because it is considered, in most cases, a minor cause or complication in the more dramatic ailments, it escapes the full attention it deserves. There is, however, nothing minor about catarrh at any time. Victims of catarrhal deafness know full well that catarrh is a serious problem. The same serious view of early or chronic catarrh would be accepted if the victim of bronchitis, colitis and cystitis realized the special part catarrh plays in these complaints.

The principal object of this booklet is the relief of the nasal and respiratory catarrh which afflicts so many people. Nonetheless, catarrh can be found in the respiratory and digestive systems simultaneously and the measures outlined to relieve nasal or respiratory catarrh will benefit the entire body and reduce catarrh in whatever part of the body it may be present.

Catarrh is an extremely common complaint. It is also no respecter of age. The early snuffles of over-fed babies and children often lay the foundation for life-long catarrh unless drastic alterations are made in the mode of life. The dietetic errors which lead to catarrh in children at a very early age are often continued through life, producing the chronic catarrh which creates so much avoidable misery. Many people are constantly afflicted with catarrh and have never experienced freedom from that state.

Irritation of any section of mucous membrane can produce catarrh. Despite the precautions against irritation of the air passages which nature provides, the nasal passages, throat and lungs are frequently still vulnerable to irritants and foreign bodies in the atmosphere. Where this is grossly polluted, as in some industrial districts and large cities, it is virtually impossible to escape some degree of irritation of the mucous membranes lining the respiratory tract.

Protection against irritation of the respiratory tract begins with the nose, which is divided by a septum into two nostrils. The fine hair in the nostrils is for the specific purpose of trapping foreign bodies and preventing their entry to the lungs.

The nasal cavities—antrums and sinuses—all play their part in warming and filtering air to guard against irritation. Infiltration of foreign bodies and irritants to the lungs is checked to a very large extent by the elaborate processes nature provides.

But nature is unable to prevent all irritation of the mucous membrane lining the respiratory tract. The more irritants are present in the atmosphere the greater the strain upon the mucous membrane—especially that of the nasal cavities and throat, which are the passages nearest to the irritants. Since they are subject to the most bombardment from irritants and are more intimately affected by temperature changes, it is not surprising that colds, nasal catarrh and other manifestations of catarrh in the head and throat areas should be common. Even to step from an over-heated room into the chilly night air can be an irritant to sensitive mucous membrane.

A simple expedient to guard against drastic changes in temperature is to place a handkerchief or thin scarf over the mouth and nose to minimize the shock of the cold air. The covering material should be gradually taken away, thus easing the transition from warm air to cold.

It is not possible to eliminate all the external irritations or thermal changes which affect mucous membranes. Nature anticipates this in providing so many precautions against irritation. However, when the irritants attack the mucous membrane, an excess of mucus is secreted and has to be discharged from the body—creating the common complaint called catarrh. The discharge of catarrh (or catarrhal mucus) from the body should not be discouraged, despite the embarrassment and discomfort it may cause. It is only by eliminating the mucus from the system and preventing the irritation which initially causes an excess of mucus in the body, that catarrh can be cured.

CHAPTER TWO

GUARDING AGAINST IRRITANTS

A VIVID illustration of the speed with which nature reacts to its environment is the coughing and spluttering which immediately arises when the head is enshrouded in pungent fumes or a cloud of dust. The delicate mucous membrane of the throat and nasal passage is irritated by the chemicals, foreign bodies or obnoxious dust and there is an immediate out-throw of mucus to ease the expulsion of the foreign material. The muscular reaction of coughing and sneezing that arises from the irritation is a reflex movement that assists the expulsion. The reaction demonstrates how nature is always striving to maintain a condition of balance or health.

Constant irritation, especially when it is severe, causes the glands in the mucous membrane to multiply and increase the supply of sputum. This is seen in chronic bronchitis, where the mucus-secreting structures grow to excess, and explains the persistent cough which is nature's attempt to eliminate the excess of mucus present in the bronchial system.

The excessive secretion of mucus is not due entirely to direct irritation. In chronic bronchitis, as in other areas where there is a long-standing catarrhal condition and subjection to irritants, glandular secretion is increased by nervous reflexes. Constant irritation, therefore, eventually increases the mucus-secreting structures, involving the nervous reflexes in the glands during the process.

With the extension or hypertrophy of the mucus-secreting system in the bronchial passages, it is not surprising that an excess of mucus, together with attempts to expel it, should be characteristic of bronchitis, especially chronic bronchitis.

Simple catarrh should not be ignored and the irritants which create catarrh should be avoided. It is impossible to eliminate all of them but it is unreasonable to expect freedom from catarrh when irritants are encouraged, for instance when tobacco in any form is smoked to excess. The 'smoker's cough' is the first indication that toxic irritants are having a deleterious effect on mucous membranes. Smoking to excess inevitably produces some degree of catarrh.

Smoking is a common example of the way irritation affects mucous membrane and of nature's attempts to relieve the condition by the characteristic cough. What should not be ignored is the less obvious effect upon the non-smoker who is in close proximity to the tobacco smoke. The irritants which attack the mucous membranes of the respiratory passages are to be found everywhere. Smoking is merely a common example.

In crowded cities, air pollution is a serious problem; inadequate ventilation of rooms, offices, factories and public transport frequently adds to the damage. Despite all attempts at setting up smokeless zones and controlling industrial smoke from factory chimneys, the streets and roads are polluted with poisonous smoke from millions of diesel and petrol engines in public and private transport. Irritants from polluted air, which is in itself a form of industrial waste, are a profound source of discomfort to millions of people.

People living in the country, away from crowded cities, have a greater degree of immunity from air pollution. Even they, however, are sometimes afflicted when intensive chemical spraying of crops or land is being carried out.

Irritants abound everywhere. The home aerosol whether it is used for domestic or personal use can be a menace to sensitive mucous membranes of the nose and throat. A mask or face covering should be used whenever an aerosol is being employed. Bathing in heavily chlorinated water, which is quite common in bathing pools, can produce a temporary irritation which sets up catarrh.

Unfortunately, much catarrh which should only be temporary and is perhaps aggravated by some irritant such as damp climate or exposure to fumes, is made worse by treating the complaint with nasal drops, inhalants or sprays. Some of the common patent medicines for catarrh, whether as drops, sprays or inhalants, damage the fine, whip-like cilia of the mucous membrane. The purpose of this cilia is to propel the flow of mucus outwards, so that it can be discharged. Any damage to it inhibits the flow of mucus, which then thickens and a nasal blockage causes stuffiness in the head and nose.

It is essential that the flow of mucus, annoying though it may be, should be uninterrupted so that blockage cannot arise to irritate the membranes even further. Constant attempts to stem the flow of mucus merely aggravate the position, and any worsening of the situation tends to convert a temporary catarrh into a chronic condition.

It must always be borne in mind when treating catarrh that the flow of mucus is merely nature's attempt to eliminate irritants and is a natural response to irritation, from any cause whatsoever, of the mucous

membrane. *Catarrh can even be regarded as a benefit
to the system when it is only a temporary condition,
for an acute attack of catarrh—as opposed to chronic
catarrh—does demonstrate nature's ability to rid itself
of the irritants which have impinged upon the mucous
membrane.*

It is for this very reason that it is important to verify
the actual cause of the catarrh and remove the cause,
or causes, rather than attempt to suppress the catarrh
by nasal drops or inhalants, etc. Constant attempts
at suppression and failure to eliminate the factors
which created the ailment only bring about a chronic
condition.

A cold is often preceded by a catarrhal condition
and should be regarded as a warning that nature is
attempting to eliminate excessive waste products of the
body. It is only when catarrh is prolonged for more than
a day or two or when the attacks are too frequent
or more severe, that serious consideration should be
given to it.

The most obvious causes of catarrh, apart from
dietary factors which will be discussed later, are as
follows:

Climatic: Dampness, lack of sun, rapid changes in
weather.

Atmospheric: Air pollution (dust, chemicals from
smoke and diesel and petrol fumes), poor ventilation.

Industrial: Occupation where fumes, dust or chemical irritants are present in excessive amounts, such
as those of foundry workers, miners, bakers, millers,
and cement workers.

Habits: Smoking, defective use of lungs, lack of
exercise and fresh air.

Not included above, but very important in the cause of catarrh, is the mistaken use of nasal drops, inhalants and sprays which I have already noted. There are also dangers from strong antiseptic gargles sometimes used in the mistaken idea that offending germs will be killed. Often the gargle is made so strong it destroys protective germs and damages the mucous membrane. In this respect gargles can be just as irritating as chlorinated swimming water.

With gradual improvement in working and living conditions, hygiene, air pollution and education, it should be possible to lessen the incidence of catarrh. The fact that this is not achieved, and that catarrh can be just as common in areas where industrial pollution is less intense, demonstrates that other factors must be taken into consideration.

It has been noted that catarrh can be found in those parts of the body where mucous membrane exists and can be irritated. Irritants therefore, are not merely those external ones which damage the respiratory system. There must be another source of irritant. This is usually found in dietetic errors and in the way food is grown and prepared.

CHAPTER THREE

DIET AND CATARRH

It is not sufficient to say that a diet must be rich in vitamins, especially vitamins A, D, and C, to avoid catarrh. When too much stress is placed upon certain vitamins, there is a tendency to concentrate on them by purchasing proprietary concoctions which contain more than the usual proportion of them. While certai͏n juice extracts and food preparations can be extreme͏. valuable, the emphasis should be on a balanced diet which contains all the vitamins and mineral salts in natural form. Any vitamin additions should only be taken to supplement the diet and, possibly, in the winter.

The growing amount of chemicals in the normal food one consumes has been a problem for years. It has reached explosion point and vast numbers of people are now seriously concerned with what can be called 'factory farming' and its effect upon world health.

It has been estimated that any of about 1,000 chemicals are introduced into food in one way or another. Little legislation has yet been produced to force manufacturers to state exactly what chemical and other additives are used in food preparation. But pressures are growing to force this issue and the legal enforcement on misrepresentation of goods and prices has helped in some directions.

Chemicals in food play a big part in diet because of their toxic, irritating and frequently accumulative nature. Some chemicals undoubtedly irritate delicate mucous membranes and are a hindrance to any potential victim of catarrh.

The mass marketing of food raises vast problems in other directions, particularly perhaps in the case of flour. White bread and white flour have long been known as deficiency foods. But a stone ground flour of around 82 per cent extraction which retains all the vitamins and mineral salts and only removes a percentage of the bran is the ideal flour for bread and confectionery.

A balanced diet is one of the main factors in producing health in the body. All the essential elements in nutrition should be freely available. Food should be consumed for enjoyment; but its main purpose is growth, repair, the production of energy and the supply of regulators and protective elements for the body.

Food is divided into protein, carbohydrates, fats, vitamins, mineral salts and water.

The carbohydrates are the cheaper 'filling' foods which, in the form of bread, cakes, pastries and other flour products, predominate in most diets. Other popular carbohydrates are sugar, rice, potatoes and macaroni and spaghetti. It is unfortunate that the best carbohydrates (wholemeal bread, whole grain rice, and other wholegrain cereals, natural sugars and honey) are neglected and that potatoes, unless served in their jackets, lose a great deal of nutriment. It is this concentration on the least nutritive carbohydrates such as white flour, white sugar and refined cereals which causes an imbalance in the diet and, because such foods are mucus-forming, tends to create catarrh.

Fats are essential to health—for energy and body

warmth. The best sources of so-called E.F.A. (essential fatty acids) are sunflower oil, corn oil and other vegetable oils. Dairy produce—milk and butter—also contain E.F.A., but meat fat is an unsatisfactory source.

Protein is found in meat, fish, eggs, cheese, nuts, etc., and a limited amount is necessary for health. Most people eat an excess of protein.

Vitamins, mineral salts and water are contained in most foods in varying degrees, but the richest sources are fresh fruit and vegetables.

The simplest formula for a balanced diet is as follows:

Protein	20 per cent
Starches, sugars and fats	20 per cent
Fruits and vegetables	60 per cent

As many of the items as possible should be in their 'whole' state, which means that as much food as possible should be in its raw state and unspoilt by cooking processes; also that, so far as possible, it should be compost grown and not produced by artificial fertilizers or contaminated with chemicals.

As much fruit as possible should be in its raw state and at least one raw salad a day should be included in the diet. A raw salad and fruit meal a day will almost automatically ensure a balanced diet and give the required vitamins and mineral salts necessary for health.

One of the important things in diet is to maintain an acid-alkali balance. Certain foods are more acid-forming than others and some foods are alkaline. An excess of acid foods tends to destroy the balance in the system and cause complaints varying from ordinary acidity to catarrh and rheumatism, etc.

Fruit and vegetables are, on the whole, alkaline, and help to maintain a healthy acid-alkali balance. There are certain exceptions to the alkaline effect on fruit in particular. A sour taste does not necessarily mean that the fruit has an acid effect in the body—citrus fruit, apples and grapes have certain acids but their effect in the body is alkaline and not acid. Some fruits do have an acid effect, but are still permitted, for example, plums and prunes. Certain foods contain oxalic acid but can still be recommended—spinach is one. Rhubarb contains so much oxalic acid it should never be used.

Balance in diet is easily maintained if sufficient fruit, vegetables and raw salads appear in the diet. A list of the common acid and alkaline foods is given below:

Acid	*Alkaline*
Meat	Root and leaf vegetables
Fish	Dried and fresh fruit
Dairy produce	(exceptions are given above)
Sugar	
Bread (white or brown)	
Flour products	
Cereals	
Fried foods	
Tea, coffee, cocoa	
Chocolate, ice-cream	

Consideration of the orthodox diet, with its stress on meat, white flour products, refined sugar, boiled-out vegetables, fried foods and tea or coffee, etc., shows how much concentration there is on acid-forming foods.

This produces an imbalance in diet that is reflected in reduced vitality and a lower resistance to disease. Under fairly normal conditions, when an imbalance in diet is neither excessive nor prolonged, the body contains sufficient safeguards to make efficient use of the food consumed, regardless of its alkaline or acid properties. Continued use of a preponderance of acid-forming foods, however, does place a strain on the body, especially the kidneys.

Health can only be experienced when the diet is balanced and all the organs of elimination are working harmoniously. Correct nutrition is vital, but oxygen, exercise and hygiene are also essential. This does mean, of course, that deep breathing is essential to make the maximum use of the lungs, and that the skin is kept in good condition by exposure to air and some daily friction and that work or exercise is necessary to burn up the fuel (food) provided.

CHAPTER FOUR

PLANNING YOUR DIET

THERE is a factor in diet which frequently provides the clue to why so many people, children and adults, continually suffer from catarrh. It is the fact that acid-forming foods also tend to create mucus. Any diet which contains an excess of these is almost sure to create a catarrhal condition.

Common Mucus-forming Foods

Bread and all cakes and pastries (especially se made
 from white flour and white sugar)
White sugar
Cereals (especially refined cereals)
White rice, spaghetti, macaroni, ravioli
Milk, cheese, butter
All fried foods
Cocoa, chocolate, ice-cream and milk puddings

It is not suggested that all acid and mucus-forming foods should be eliminated from the diet to relieve catarrh, although it is possible to completely curtail them for a short period every so often to rid the body of an accumulation of catarrh. The best plan is to balance the diet by placing greater emphasis on the alkaline elements and by choosing the most nutritious of the mucus-forming foods.

Wholewheat bread and wholewheat cakes or biscuits are obviously better than bread or cakes produced from devitalized white flour. Unrefined sugar is less concentrated and possesses the natural properties which are removed from refined white sugar.

The best cereals are compost-grown oatmeal, natural (brown) rice, buckwheat and breakfast cereals with a wholewheat or bran origin. Cottage cheese is superior to most cheeses and processed cheese is the least desirable.

Home-made ice-cream is preferable to the factory-made product. Even so the consumption of ice-cream should be severely curtailed. Fried foods should be completely avoided. Cocoa is definitely not a good drink for any catarrh sufferer. Chocolate sweets or bars are very concentrated and should be severely curtailed if catarrh is to be overcome.

There is no need to make the diet unattractive to cure catarrh. The child who is allowed too much fried food, white bread, pastries, cakes, milk puddings, chocolates, sweets and ice-cream is almost certain to suffer from catarrh. If this unbalanced system of feeding is perpetuated into later life a whole host of physical ailments with catarrh a prominent feature are certain to be encountered. It is essential, therefore, that correct feeding should begin at a very early age. Nor is this so difficult as may be imagined. There are very few children who will not delight in chewing a fresh raw carrot; these, along with with apples, oranges and other fruits are not used enough in ordinary households to counter a natural, but fostered, demand for chocolates and other sweets.

It is possible to completely forego all mucus-forming foods for short periods, so that the accumulation of catarrh and other toxic waste matter that accumulates in the system can be eliminated. Knowing that mucus-forming foods almost inevitably spring from the acid

group of foods, to cleanse the system it is obvious
that the eliminative diet will be based on the alkaline
elements in food.

The most efficient and at the same time most drastic
method of quickly clearing catarrh is to fast for a few
days on grapes or oranges or clear vegetable soup or
fruit juices, or on a combination of them. To exist on
oranges or other fruit and drinks only is not real
fasting and few people are incapable of undergoing
such a regime. It should be attempted for one day only
on the first occasion and then can be repeated at weekly
intervals. If the catarrh is very obstinate this process
may have to be repeated over several weeks; by that
time the average person will have discovered that three
days of such 'fasting' is a feasible proposition to
accelerate the cure.

For those who are unable or unwilling to embark
on the very strict regimen, the following eliminative
diet is the next logical step. The ideal process would
be to have two days of 'fasting' and then commence
the eliminative diet outlined below:—

On rising	Diluted fruit juice.
Breakfast	Fruit only. (Choose three from any of the following: oranges, apples, grapes, raisins, prunes, figs, dates). Fruit drink or 1 cup weak tea if desired.
Mid-morning	Cup of Marmite or dandelion coffee or glass of fruit juice.
Lunch	Fresh or dried fruit (not rhubarb or tinned fruit). Small salad of lettuce, tomato and raw grated carrot. Oil and lemon or cider vinegar dressing.

Tea	Cup of weak tea or Marmite or fruit juice.
Supper	As lunch. The salad can be slightly varied according to season: *e.g.*, celery, tomato and watercress and raw carrot or endive, tomato, onion and carrot.
Last thing	Apple or grape juice or Marmite or Vecon.

The above diet is free from mucus-forming foods and is very alkaline and, therefore, an eliminating diet. The reaction from this diet may at first appear to be far from desirable. It is more than probable that *more, not less* catarrh will be present.

The fact that the diet may appear to aggravate rather than lessen the symptoms is due to the emphasis on elimination in the diet and an expected indication that the inherent healing powers of the body are stimulated to the extent of expelling the mucus accumulated in the system. It is only by reducing the formation of mucus and stimulating the expulsion of waste products that an acid-alkali balance can be achieved and the catarrh dispelled. In the cleansing process involved in the eliminative diet it is anticipated that, for a short period, the symptoms may be worse.

The eliminative diet can be carried out in several variations, according to circumstances. The most effective plan is to exist on it for a clear week. It can, however, be undertaken for just one or two days a week, being repeated at weekly intervals for a period of anything from one to three months. Even under normal circumstances it is a good plan to prevent illness by having an 'elimination day' at least once a month.

To undertake the elimination diet is only part of the

process. It is obviously essential to correct the imbalance in normal feeding, so that an excess of the normal mucus-forming is avoided. It is in connection with normal diet that anomalies can be found. Some people have a greater disposition to catarrh than others. To some extent this can be attributed to factors such as smoking, environment, faulty oxidation of the blood-stream (often due to shallow breathing and badly ventilated rooms), central heating, lack of exercise and *to a lowered tolerance to mucus-forming foods*.

There appears to be a certain category of person who is unable to tolerate the quantity of normal mucus-forming materials which the average person can accept. An awareness of this tolerance factor is a personal matter, and this type of person must reduce mucus-forming food intake to his or her particular level. This, fortunately, can be achieved without creating a deficiency diet.

This 'tolerance factor' is an explanation of why, for instance, some people can exist on a diet which is relatively low in mucus-forming foods and still suffer from a mild degree of catarrh while others under the same conditions are completely free of catarrh.

Normal Menus for Catarrh

Example 1:

On rising	1 glass diluted fruit juice.
Breakfast	2 thin slices wholemeal toast, butter and honey. Stewed prunes or raisins or apples, Froment or Bemax with yogurt or fruit juice or muesli.
Mid-morning	Weak tea or coffee or Marmite or Vecon.

Lunch	Steamed or grilled fish.
	Potatoes or swede and one green vegetable.
	Baked apple or pears or melon.
Tea	Weak tea or diluted fruit juice only.
Supper	2-3 Ryvita or similar biscuits and butter.
	Raw salad with cottage cheese or hard-boiled egg or cold meat or onion soup.
	Fresh apple or orange or grapes.
Last thing	Dandelion coffee or diluted fruit juice.

Example 2:

On rising	As 1.
Breakfast	As 1.
Mid-morning	As 1.
Lunch	Lamb or mutton or veal (grilled or casseroled).
	Grilled tomatoes with spinach or greens.
	Carrots or leeks or onions.
	Fresh fruit.
Tea	Weak tea or diluted fruit juice.
Supper	2-3 Ryvita or similar biscuits and butter.
	Baked potato or baked chestnuts.
	Raw salad with cottage cheese.
	Fresh fruit or prunes and yogurt.
Last thing	As 1.

Example 3:

On rising	As 1.
Breakfast	As 1: a boiled or poached egg may be added.

Mid-morning	As 1.
Lunch	Rice dish with tomatoes, etc.
	Beetroot or red cabbage or cauliflower.
	Spinach or celery or leeks.
	Baked apple or stewed pears and yogurt.
Tea	As 1.
Supper	2-3 Ryvita or similar biscuits and butter.
	Salad (with apple, raisins, or grapes etc.) and cottage cheese.
	Cold meat or sardines or onion soup.
	Apple or melon or grapes.
Last thing	As 1.

Example 4:

On rising	As 1.
Breakfast	As 1.
Mid-morning	As 1.
Lunch	Stewed steak or minced meat with onions, carrots and tomatoes and small potato.
	Swede or parsnip or greens.
	Fruit jelly (made with fruit and Gellozone).
Tea	As 1.
Supper	2-3 Ryvita or similar biscuits.
	Baked potato with cheese centre.
	Raw salad.
	Yogurt mixed with dates and raisins.
Last thing	As 1.

Example 5:

On rising	As 1.
Breakfast	As 1.
Mid-morning	Dandelion coffee or Marmite or Vecon.
Lunch	Onion or leek *au gratin* and grilled tomatoes.

	Baked or steamed potato and carrots. Stewed apricots or figs.
Tea	As 1.
Supper	2-3 Ryvita or similar biscuits and butter.
	Mushrooms or cold meat.
	Salad,
	Fresh fruit and yogurt.
Last thing	Marmite or Vecon or dandelion coffee or fruit juice.

Example 6:

On rising	As 1.
Breakfast	As 1, with egg if desired.
Mid-morning	As 1.
Lunch	Steamed or grilled fish with potato.
	Carrots or leeks or greens and a tomato salad.
	Baked apple or stewed pears.
Tea	As 1.
Supper	Onion soup.
	2-3 Ryvita or similar biscuits and butter.
	Cottage cheese salad.
	Prunes or raisins or dates and yogurt.
Last thing	Diluted tomato juice or fruit juice or dandelion coffee.

Example 7:

On rising	As 1.
Breakfast	As 1.
Mid-morning	As 1.
Lunch	Chicken or veal or lamb with grilled tomatoes.
	Onion or leeks and celery or greens.
	Fruit jelly or baked banana.

Tea	As 1.
Supper	2-3 Ryvita or similar biscuits and butter.
	Baked potato or baked chestnuts or cold meat.
	Salad.
	Yogurt with fresh fruit salad.
Last thing	As 1.

Example 8:

On rising	As 1.
Breakfast	As 1.
Mid-morning	As 1.
Lunch	Meat and vegetable stew or stewed lamb chops or liver with onions and carrots and barley.
	Cauliflower or greens with swede or parsnip.
	Baked or stewed apple.
Tea	As 1.
Supper	Onion soup.
	2-3 Ryvita or similar biscuits and butter.
	Salad with hard-boiled egg.
	Fresh fruit and yogurt.
Last thing	Vegetable broth or dandelion coffee or diluted fruit juice.

The above examples are a guide to what a balanced diet should present on the table. Recipes will be found in the next chapter. For those who do not eat meat, suitable vegetarian savouries will be listed.

The diet shows very little bread, but where Ryvita biscuits are mentioned any similar biscuit or oatmeal biscuit will be just as acceptable. Two thin slices of wholemeal toast can replace the biscuits.

There is no reason why the meals should stay in the order given. If it is easier to have a salad lunch and a cooked meal at night, then the order can be reversed, but one salad and fruit meal per day is essential.

The onion family—onions, leeks, garlic and olives are very beneficial in the relief of catarrh and should be used extensively in the diet. Chives make a welcome addition to salads and it is possible to obtain garlic in capsule form as well as in its natural state.

A valuable addition to the main meals is a small glass of raw vegetable juice. This is especially important for those who are unable to digest a lot of raw food. A very tasty raw drink can be made from equal parts of raw carrot, beetroot and apple juice. Children usually enjoy this drink and the raw beetroot juice gives a pleasant colour to the drink. The juice should be regarded as a food and *sipped slowly* to gain the maximum advantage.

Raw vegetable and fruit juices can be bought at any good health food store if a liquidizer is not available. It should be pointed out, too, that the diluted fruit juices can be bottled or canned provided they are unsweetened and natural. Fruit squashes are not recommended.

One of the advantages of eating raw salads and fruit is that they do demand thorough mastication. Meals should be enjoyed and food should be thoroughly chewed before swallowing and this does mean that sufficient time should be allowed for meals. Thorough mastication ensures the maximum benefit from food and reduces the temptation to over-eat—in fact it will be observed that health is generally improved by eating less but chewing it more. A balanced diet, therefore, when properly masticated will, in time, tend to make an obese person slimmer while a thin person will gain weight.

Where food is cooked, as far as possible it should be baked, grilled, steamed, casseroled or pressure-cooked or cooked conservatively. The latter means by using very, very little water and refers more to green vegetables. The liquid left over from conservative cooking in particular is valuable for making vegetable broth or soup or sauces. A little Marmite or Yeastrel or tomato juice added to the vegetable liquid makes a pleasant and nourishing drink. One last word on cooking is that aluminium pans are the least desirable cooking utensils and should never be used for acid fruit.

Food, as well as maintaining health, should be enjoyed. The real flavour of food can best be appreciated in many cases when it is either in its natural raw state or cooked without being ruined in masses of boiling water which detract from its natural goodness and destroy its flavour. Use as little water as possible in cooking and find out what a different flavour vegetables possess, while the vitamins and mineral salts will not be entirely destroyed and thrown down the drain.

Another point when cooking or serving food is that condiments should be used sparingly. Excessive use of condiments spoils the natural flavour of food and irritates the mucous membranes of the digestive tract— and can help to cause catarrh. On the whole, table condiments should be avoided. A little salt can be used with eggs and the salad dressing should be limited to olive or sunflower oil and cider vinegar or lemon juice. Cooked vegetables and baked potatoes are often improved by the addition of a little oil, which is a healthy substitute for butter or condiments.

CHAPTER FIVE

RECIPES FOR CATARRH SUFFERERS

THE following recipes are designed to reduce the mucus-forming element in the diet. It is neither possible, advisable nor even necessary to completely eliminate all mucus or acid-forming foods from the normal diet; such an objective can only be achieved in the strict therapeutic elimination diet or fasting. The recipes, therefore, do employ limited quantities of mucus-forming food, but are still consistent with health and relative or complete freedom from catarrh.

Muesli: Can be used as a breakfast food or as a sweet with lunch or supper. It is very simple to make and can be varied by using any fruit that is to hand.

1 tablespoon coarse oatmeal soaked overnight in

3 tablespoons of water.

In the morning add

1 coarsely grated Bramley apple,

grated lemon or orange rind,

1 dessertspoon of milled cashew nuts and

1 dessertspoon of nut cream or top of milk.

Mix well together and serve.

Bramley apple is recommended for the flavour, which goes well with muesli and its economy, but any apple can be used. Prunes, figs, sultanas, raisins, dates or grapefruit can be equally well used in a muesli, or even a combination of fresh or dried fruit, according to taste.

Yogurt: Can be used in many variations apart from being served plain. Fruit, especially grapes, bananas, orange and grapefruit segments and raisins, mix well with yogurt. When served as a savoury, yogurt and thin slices of cucumber make an excellent summer dish. Mixed with thin slices of onion, chopped or sliced peppers and a few herbs, yogurt can be served separately or on salads.

Soups: Can play an important part in a diet for catarrh.

Potato and Onion Soup: Slice 2 large or 3 medium onions into rings and cook slowly in ½ pint water with a little milk or vegetable stock added. When the onions are half cooked, coarsely grate an equal quantity of washed (unpeeled) potato into the onions. Add a little seasoning to taste, but salt should be used with discretion. Marvel or fat-free milk could be used in all the soups.

Potato and Leek Soup: Can be made in the same manner, leeks being sliced into thin rings rather than lengthways.

Celery and Onion Soup: Another favourite which varies the onion theme. Onions and the onion family are essential to catarrhal people and should be served as frequently as possible. Both the celery and the onion should be cooked in slices—quarter of a celery and two large onions. When the celery and onions are partly cooked, add 2 medium washed potatoes grated on a coarse grater. Season to taste.

Cheese: There are any number of recipes containing cheese which, it must be admitted, does add protein and taste to diet. People with a predisposition to catarrh, however, are advised to use less cheese than the normal individual. However, there is still no reason why cheese dishes should be excluded, providing the cheese is well balanced by vegetables, particularly onions and leeks, etc.

To make feeding a little more interesting, there is no reason why celery, cauliflower, marrow, aubergine or mushrooms should not be added to the leeks or onions in an *au gratin* dish.

Seaweed: Extracts like Gellozone, Agar-agar and Carrageen Moss are beneficial to catarrh and should be employed as thickening agents instead of flour when making a sauce. The method is as follows:

Mix 2 teaspoons of Gellozone with a little vegetable stock or fat-free milk. Add ½ pint of boiling vegetable stock over a low flame or burner, until dissolved. A larger quantity of Gellozone will make the sauce thicker, if desired. Add the grated cheese (sufficient to give a good cheese flavour), season to taste with herbs and salt and pour over the cooked onions or leeks, with any different vegetables that are added.

Conventional Sauce: If a conventional sauce is really preferred, in which flour is used, then it should be made with fat-free milk, vegetable stock or tomato juice and wholemeal (not white) flour. The following is a quick and easy method of preparing a sauce:

4 tablespoons wholemeal flour.
1 ounce butter or vegetable margarine.
½ pint fat-free milk, vegetable water or tomato juice.
Mix the flour with sufficient of the liquid to produce a thin paste. Heat the remaining liquid and bring it to boiling point. While boiling, pour in the flour mixture

slowly, stirring all the time. Boil for a few seconds, stirring all the time, and add the grated cheese and seasoning to taste. Should the sauce appear "lumpy", pour through a strainer onto the cooked vegetables.

Vegetarian dishes: These need not be dull; indeed many are far from it. A lot of stews can be made with no meat at all, yet be very tasty.

Aubergine Stew: Slice 2 large or 3 medium onions into rings and cook in little water. When almost cooked, add slices of aubergine (or cucumber), sliced tomatoes, a few chopped mushrooms, 2 tablespoons of grated cheese, a pinch of herbs and salt to taste. Place in a casserole and finish cooking in the oven.

Bean Stew: Cook 4 ounces butter beans and the same quantity of onions or leeks till almost quite soft, then add 8 ounces of sliced tomato, 4 ounces grated cheese, herbs and salt to taste and cook in the oven for a further 20 minutes. The beans and onions should be cooked in as little water as possible. Carrots or celery could be added to the beans and onions for variety.

A similar dish can be produced by using lentils instead of butter beans.

Brown Rice: Ordinary white rice should never be given to victims of catarrh. The conventional rice pudding made with white rice, milk and white sugar is a very mucus-forming dish. Natural, brown rice, however, can be used to make savoury dishes. One way to use it is thus:

Wash 2 tablespoons of brown rice and cook for 30 minutes in a double boiler, using vegetable stock, Marmite or Yeastrel or tomato juice. More liquid may be required as the rice cooks and swells.

Slice or coarsely grate two or three of the following vegetables: onions, leeks, celery, carrot, red or green peppers, mushrooms. Cook in a little oil and water, adding herbs and salt to taste.

The rice should be soft and separate easily when cooked. Add the cooked vegetables to the rice and mix together. Place one layer of the rice mixture in a casserole, followed by a thin layer of grated cheese and then another layer of rice mixture. Cover with a layer of thinly sliced tomatoes and cook for a few minutes.

Nut Mixture: Almost the same procedure can be adopted, producing a different flavour, by using milled cashew nuts instead of brown rice. In this case the vegetables should be diced (or sliced into rings) and cooked in a little oil and water. When the vegetables are cooked, stir in the milled nuts and a little grated cheese and place in a greased dish. Cover the mixture with sliced tomatoes and cook in a low oven for 30 minutes.

The nut mixture, as above, is ideal as a stuffing for other vegetables—marrow, aubergine, potato, onion, pepper or tomato. Some of the inside of the onion or tomato can be used in the stuffing. A recommended way of cooking onions, either for stuffing or for general use, is to bake them in the oven in the natural state, unpeeled.

It is possible to produce a very simple meal by just having baked potato and baked onion together with a poached or scrambled egg. Instead of having butter with the potato, sunflower oil can be most satisfactory and is infinitely superior from a dietetic and health point of view. Oil, in fact, should not be reserved for salads; most cooked vegetables can be improved by the addition of a little sunflower or olive oil instead of condiments.

Salads: These can be improvised all the year round and should not be confined to lettuce and tomato and, possibly, spring onions or cucumber. Salads should be made as varied as possible and adapted to the particular time of year. It is better, and more economical, to use the vegetables and salad foods that are in season rather than buy expensive out-of-season foods. In any case, *forced* lettuces and other greenstuffs do not have the same flavour or food value as the products of the season. Chopping cabbage, red or green, and celery are much better buys in the winter.

There are so many items from which salads can be produced all the year round that no salad should ever be unattractive or lack colour. Salad foods include:

Lettuce, watercress, cress, endive, chicory, red or green cabbage, nasturtiums, carrots, raw and cooked beetroot, raw cauliflower, tomato, onion, leek, radish, cucumber, swede, celeriac, peppers and the herbs: parsley, mint, thyme, chives, garlic.

Additions to raw salads can include hard boiled eggs, sardines and pilchards, cold meat, cottage or lactic cheese, raisins, grapes, dates, nuts, slices of apple, pineapple or melon, segments of orange or grapefruit and even stewed prunes. Cooked potato or sweetcorn is often included in a salad.

A conventional salad can be made from lettuce, tomato, raw grated carrot, cooked or raw beetroot, slices of onion or leek and decorated with sprigs of raw cauliflower, a little hard boiled egg or cheese and some slices of red or green pepper. Segments of orange, a couple of prunes or slices of melon can add a touch of colour.

A winter salad can be produced by using thinly shredded red or green cabbage. Mix a coarsely grated Bramley apple and a few rings of leek or onion into the cabbage together with oil and cider vinegar and a little dried parsley. The cabbage should be prepared two hours before the meal, if possible, and, before serving, decorate it with slices of carrot, cooked beetroot, sprigs of cauliflower, pieces of cheese and slices of orange or melon.

Fruit goes well with a salad. It can always be used either for decoration or even as a base. A salad made with lettuce or watercress, tomato, grated carrot and beetroot can have, as a centre piece, a yogurt mixture of yogurt and any fruit that is at hand. Slices of banana, apple, grapes and raisins can be mixed into the yogurt.

There are times when vegetables are profuse and reasonably cheap. Cooked runner beans with thin slices of tomato, rings of onion and raw grated carrot or beetroot make another useful base for salads. Oil, cider vinegar and a few herbs should be added to the runner bean mixture. For a change, such a salad can be decorated with sardines, asparagus or cold meat, sprigs of raw cauliflower or nasturtium, cress and a little grated or cottage cheese.

Potato salad is an obvious base, but it should always have onion or leek included and plenty of raw salad material should always be served with it. It is the raw food that is the most important and most beneficial.

Packed lunch: For the thousands of people who have to eat out at lunchtime there is no reason why a salad and fruit lunch cannot be packed. On the whole, salads are increasing in popularity, both in restaurants and canteens. Where there is difficulty in obtaining a suitable meal, the excellent food containers now available make packed meals really possible.

A suitable packed lunch could be:

4 Ryvita or crispbread biscuits and butter.

Hard boiled egg or cold meat or cottage cheese.

Lettuce, endive or watercress, tomato, slices of raw celery or carrot and sprigs of raw cauliflower.

Apple and raisins or ripe banana and dates or other fruit in season.

The above meal requires little preparation and is infinitely superior to a *commercial* meal of fried food and boiled-out vegetables or even, as in some cases, re-heated food.

It must be reiterated that food should be a pleasure. Meals should look good and taste good. The distinctive flavour of food is being lost by the modern methods of food production. Compost grown vegetables possess the best flavour, but they must be served raw or be steamed, casseroled, grilled or baked to preserve the flavour. Nor must that flavour be ruined by condiments, many of which are irritants to the delicate mucous membrane.

A diet for catarrh can retain the pleasure in food. What is more, it can restore the sense of taste and smell (lost to many catarrhal people) which should be associated with good food.

It is not too difficult to overcome catarrh once the lessons of diet and sensible living are absorbed. Time must be allowed for the process. Chronic catarrh does not arise overnight—it is normally the result of years of dubious feeding and detrimental environment and habits. Relief of catarrh, therefore, should not be expected overnight. The definite fact is that it is possible to make catarrh just a bad memory, but it is the responsibility of the individual to keep himself (or herself) free from catarrh.

CHAPTER SIX

HOME TREATMENT FOR CATARRH

Any treatment for catarrh will have its value largely nullified if serious attempts are not made to correct the diet. At the same time the benefits of dieting can be considerably enhanced if other measures are adopted.

Diet will maintain the acid-alkali balance in the body at its correct level without imposing a strain on the system. A balanced diet will contain just the correct amount of roughage and laxative material to encourage healthy bowel function. Also, by limiting the amount of acid and mucus-forming material (reducing the protein content at the same time) it will discourage the accumulation of mucus, irritants, uric acid, urates and other waste products which poison the bloodstream and create diseases of all types.

Elimination of waste products from the body is carried out by the bowels, kidneys, lungs and skin. The diet encourages bowel action and reduces the load on the kidneys. The next step is to augment the work of the diet by encouraging lung and skin activity, so that elimination of waste matter is maintained at the peak of efficiency.

Physical effort is involved in deep breathing and in care of the skin and this, in turn, gives an impetus to the blood circulation and the passage of nutriment to the tissues and cells and the transportation of waste products from those tissues and cells.

The function of the lungs is to provide oxygen to the bloodstream and remove the carbon dioxide from the blood, which has previously circulated through the body. In normal circumstances people breathe in and out about sixteen times a minute, taking in a supply of oxygen and passing it on to the tissues through the bloodstream; at the same time the blood collects carbon dioxide which is given out by the lungs. Inspired air—the air that is drawn into the lungs—contains five per cent more oxygen than the air which is expelled from the lungs. Expired air contains four per cent more carbon dioxide than inspired air. It is only by efficient breathing that the blood can be properly oxygenated and carbon dioxide expelled.

Nasal catarrh is probably the commonest form and is quite frequently just a passing symptom and a normal reaction to irritants or a cold or damp or change in temperature. Bronchial catarrh is a result of continued subjection to irritants and an excess of mucus-forming elements in the diet. In both cases some difficulty is experienced in breathing and it is all-important to learn to breathe correctly, even at a very early age, making the maximum use of the lungs as well as freeing the air passages of mucus.

Correct breathing: Deep breathing is essential if efficient elimination of waste products from the body is to be ensured. All the tissues and nerves require the oxygen that is transported by the bloodstream. Obese people should note that oxygen is essential to burn up excess fat and that energy is dependent upon oxygen. At the same time, deep breathing removes the waste carbon dioxide.

Correct breathing must begin at the earliest possible age. The snuffles in children, which betray a catarrhal tendency, can be eliminated if the diet is correct and breathing exercises are introduced. Diaphragmatic breathing should be taught at an early age and should be practised by every victim of catarrh. Time and patience are required to master the art but, once learnt, the advantages are all too apparent.

One of the best ways to practise diaphragmatic breathing is to lie on the floor with the head slightly raised on a pillow, with the knees slightly raised. Place a book on the abdomen. On expiration the book should sink down as the abdominal muscles contract. By placing a hand on the book and pushing it down into the abdomen, the abdominal muscles can be educated to contract during expiration. On inspiration, the book should rise as the abdomen rises with inspiration. With the next expiration the book should sink again as the abdominal muscles contract.

The exercise should be augmented by additional training in front of a mirror. Either strip to the waist or wear very light clothing. Stand in front of the mirror with the hands on each side of the lower ribs, the tips of the fingers pointing towards the centre line of the front of the chest.

Begin the exercise with gentle inspiration through the nose, then noisily out through the mouth, emptying the lungs as much as possible. At the same time the fingertips should close together in the centre of the chest. Almost at the end of expiration gentle pressure should be exerted by the palms of the hands on the sides of the chest. Inspiration through the nose follows the expiration and during this the lower ribs should move outwards against the palms of the hands, forcing the fingertips apart.

Before the breathing exercises blow the nose and make sure the nasal passages are as clear as possible. To gain the best results from breathing it is necessary to relax as much as possible. This state can be assisted by a few simple exercises such as shrugging the shoulders, allowing the arms to go as limp as possible, and making a few relaxed swinging movements of the spine.

Skin treatment: It is important also that skin activity should be maintained at a high peak of efficiency and there are obvious advantages in combining relaxation exercises, skin treatment and breathing exercises in one effort.

A practical plan is to use the bathroom as a focal point and start with a good friction of the skin with a coarse towel which has been dipped into cold water. The skin should be thoroughly rubbed and a glowing effect attained. The coarsest towel possible produces the best effect.

The skin friction will increase blood circulation and automatically encourage deeper breathing and a sense of relaxation. Further relaxation can be induced by the simple exercises and then it is possible to proceed to the breathing exercises (or education of the lungs) with the knowledge that a sound basis has been laid.

Only a few minutes are involved and the amount of mucus that can be eliminated in that time and the sense of well-being created, encourages further efforts in this direction. While first thing in the morning is the best time to carry out the procedure there are concrete advantages for doing it both morning and evening.

Water treatment: Hydropathic treatments can stimulate and tone the skin and at the same time increase lung activity and the circulation of body fluids. Quite simple baths can be transformed into effective water treatments by the intelligent use of hot and cold water.

The aim of all water treatments is to dissolve and eliminate toxic matter, to improve the circulation and to strengthen the constitution. The basic rule in hydrotheraphy is that of *action and reaction*.

Applying any form of heat to the skin draws blood to the surface. It is only a transient effect, since the blood must return to the deeper tissues from which it was derived. A short cold application has this effect. By drawing the blood into the superficial tissues by applying hot water, then forcing it back into the tissues with cold, there is "push-and-pull" stimulation of blood circulation.

It is upon this basis of "action and reaction" that water treatments are based, the ultimate result of which is the dissolving and removal of waste products and the strengthening of the constitution.

Water treatments can be simple and many variations can be produced, providing the main rules are borne in mind. These rules are that hot water is enervating, cold water is stimulating and tepid water is relaxing. Over-stimulation leads to depression, and cold water, therefore, has to be used in short, sharp sessions.

Hot baths, with the addition of pine oil, are very beneficial to catarrh if a quick, cold shower follows. After any hot bath (a hot bath is over blood heat and normally about 110° C), a quick cold shower should be taken. A cold shower is not essential. A *quick* cold splash in cold water will produce the same effect.

It is vitally important that the reaction from a cold shower or plunge is that of warmth. If this is not obtained it will be because either the cold plunge lasted too long, or the person taking the cold plunge is too weak and lacks the vital energy necessary to obtain the necessary reaction. In the latter case, the water should have the chill removed from it and the duration should be shortened till enough energy is restored.

Pine oil is useful in a bath when breathing is difficult. When obesity and rheumatism are just as much a problem as catarrh the addition of 2 cups of soda or commercial Epsom salts will assist elimination of waste products. These baths, which can be almost sweating treatments, should only be taken at night, just before retiring.

Another very simple water treatment is the "salt glow". All that is required is a basin of common salt. Stand in the bath and, by continuously wetting the hands and picking up the salt, the skin can be rubbed with the wet salt. The "salt glow" should be followed by an ordinary warm bath and a cold shower and it is one of the most effective means of improving skin activity.

Steam treatment: Where the victim of catarrh possesses the necessary vitality sauna baths are strongly advised. The hot vapour of the sauna room creates profuse sweating and loosens the mucus in the lungs, making it easier to breathe. A sauna, however, is a very drastic treatment and should only be taken after advice from a medical or naturopathic practitioner.

A very simple, safe and effective way of easing the lungs and nasal passages and stimulating the removal of mucus is by ordinary steam. This can be achieved by a steam kettle—even the ordinary kitchen kettle will suffice—or by bending over a bowl of very hot water with a large towel over the head and shoulders to contain the steam in a makeshift tent. The steam should be directed at the chest, mouth and nose to penetrate the passages and loosen the mucus. Here again the best results are obtained when the surface area which has been subjected to the steam is well splashed with cold water.

Children and old people can be given the steam treatment for up to 20 minutes at a time. Bending over a bowl of very hot water is probably the safest method but, under supervision, a steam kettle should be perfectly safe. With children, or where the skin is very delicate, it is advisable to rub the area which is to be steamed with olive oil before starting.

Postural drainage: Another treatment which can help in bronchial catarrh is postural drainage. As a general rule personal guidance and education should be sought to ascertain the correct procedure for postural drainage in each particular case. What can be tried is to lean right over a bed with the arms and shoulders resting comfortably on two pillows on the floor. A chair with pillows can be similarly adapted. In this case the person would stand on the floor and bend over the chair in an inverted V fashion.

Postural drainage has to be approached gradually. It is essential to begin with 1 minute two or three times a day and only gradually increase both the duration and frequency of the treatment. Where there is a condition of long-standing and chronic bronchial catarrh, postural drainage is most effective. At the same time it can relieve distress in breathing in short-lived acute bronchial catarrh.

Skilled treatment and advice: This booklet has so far concentrated on what is possible in the relief of catarrh by diet and home treatment. This does not, however, exclude the necessity for skilled advice or treatment from a qualified naturopathic practitioner or osteopath or chiropractor.

Catarrh does not necessarily arise just from wrong diet, poor environment or faulty habits. Postural and other defects may influence and aggravate the condition. Chronic catarrh, whatever form it takes, should be regarded as a serious ailment and expert advice should be sought.

Most trained naturopaths are also osteopaths or skilled in other manipulative therapies and can give personal advice on diet and correct postural or spinal defects which do have a bearing on the catarrh. Even catarrhal deafness can often be assisted by the diet and manipulative therapies.

Manipulation will relax tension, break down and remove obstruction to the circulatory system and increase spinal mobility.

Where necessary, practitioners will give instruction in the re-education of the respiratory system by breathing exercises and in postural drainage.

Physical treatment, plus diet and the avoidance of the irritants which are known to be connected with catarrh, are measures which are far superior to drugs, nor have they such side-effects. Extremely safe, they benefit the whole system.